Sarah's Battle

How an undetected appendix resulted in septic shock

Jaylen Fleming

All rights reserved. No part of this publication may be reproduced, distributed, or transmitted in any form or by any means, including photocopying, recording, or other electronic or mechanical methods, without the prior written permission of the publisher, except in the case of brief quotations embodied in critical reviews and certain other noncommercial uses permitted by copyright law.

Copyright © Jaylen Fleming, 2024

Table of Content

Why I Wrote This Book

Introduction

Chapter One
Initial symptoms and her decision to go to the hospital

Chapter Two
The Fight for Life : Intensive care in the intensive care unit

Chapter Three
Transition from critical condition to gradual recovery

Chapter Four
Psychological impact of the experience

Chapter Five
Adoption of a Healthier Lifestyle

Chapter Six
Impact of her story on others and her role as an advocate

Chapter Seven
Reflection on her Journey and the Lessons Learned

About the Author

Why I Wrote This Book

I wrote this book to provide more clarity on septic shock, a dangerous and frequently misdiagnosed disease. My own encounter with this potentially fatal illness while working as a medical professional made me acutely aware of how little others know about it. Along the way, I faced the emotional and psychological challenges that come with experiencing something as terrible as this. In addition to the severe physical challenges.

This book is a monument to the human spirit's tenacity and the strength of willpower, hope, and support. By telling this tale, I want to reassure and counsel anyone who might be going through something similar. My goal is to provide survivors, caregivers, and families with a ray of hope by demonstrating that even with extreme difficulty, recovery is achievable.

This book also seeks to educate readers about septic shock and to emphasize the vital significance of early detection and timely medical attention. By educating people, I want to improve other people's lives and start a larger discussion about this deadly yet hidden illness. In the end, "The Journey of a Septic Shock Survivor" is a celebration of the medical experts who give their all to save lives and a reminder that hope and fortitude can be found even in the worst of circumstances.

Introduction

Living in the suburbs with her devoted husband James and their two small children, Liam and Sophie, was 32-year-old Sarah. Sarah was a committed mother and career-driven worker who managed her busy schedule as a marketing manager. She loved to run, frequently competing in regional marathons and going on family hikes on the weekends. Sarah, who was well-known for her endless vitality and upbeat outlook, relished every second of her life and her responsibilities as an athlete and caretaker. She had no idea that her life would soon take an unexpected and difficult turn..

Chapter One

Initial symptoms and her decision to go to the hospital

Sarah Peterson had always embodied vigor and health. She was a devoted wife to her husband, James, and mother to two small children, Liam and Sophie, at the age of thirty-two. She lived in a peaceful suburb and skillfully combined her busy lifestyle as an active person with her job as a marketing manager. Her weekends were occupied with soccer matches, family outings, and lively neighborhood runs. She frequently started her mornings with these activities. Sarah was the kind of person that everyone flocked toward because of her contagious energy and upbeat outlook. She also treasured every second of her busy life.

Sarah saw a sense of something wrong on a normal Tuesday morning. She awoke with a heavy lethargy that seemed to cling to her and an unsettling sense of tiredness. She first wrote it off as a result of her hectic weekend. Her family had hiked the trails of a nearby national park during the day, and she had just finished a ten-kilometer run. Sarah was used to physical exertion, but this tiredness seemed different, deeper, more ingrained.

She felt a twinge in her muscles as she struggled to get out of bed—like she had the flu. She dismissed it, got dressed, and went downstairs to make her family's breakfast. The morning ritual was well underway, with the youngsters already awake. James questioned, "You okay, Em? " after observing her lethargic motions. You seem a little strange today. She said with a comforting smile, "I'm fine." Simply worn out. Probably went overboard this past weekend. Everything went as normal for breakfast, but Sarah noticed that she was eating less than normal. It was unusual for her to lack hunger as she usually relished her early meals. As she kissed James and the kids goodbye and prepared to head to work, a faint chill ran down her spine, despite the warm summer morning.

The dull aching had become worse by the time Sarah got to the office. Her body temperature seemed to swing between waves of heat and chills, and her head felt heavy. She managed to get through her morning meetings, but her focus faltered. Sarah, who is usually clear-headed and articulate, was having trouble concentrating on the duties at hand. She made the decision to go outside for coffee in the middle of the morning, thinking the caffeine would help her return to her normal self. She felt a sense of vertigo when she was waiting in line at the café.

Breathing deeply, she steadied herself against the counter. "This is not how things usually work," she told herself. She dismissed it nonetheless, determined to get through the day.

Sarah felt her enthusiasm dwindle back at her desk. Even small chores became overwhelming, and she found herself constantly checking the time, mentally calculating the number of hours until she could return home and relax. She realized by midday that she had to stop ignoring the symptoms. Her skin was extremely sensitive to touch, her joints hurt, and she felt feverish. During lunch, Sarah made the decision to phone her doctor's office.

After hearing her list of symptoms, the receptionist encouraged her to schedule an appointment for a check-up. The receptionist remarked, "It's better to get it checked out, but it could be the flu." Sarah accepted, but she made the decision to go to the doctor after finishing her employment. She was careful not to appear overly dramatic.. However, as the afternoon progressed, her condition worsened. She felt lightheaded and noticed that her heart was racing even while she was sitting still. The chills became more intense, and she couldn't get warm no matter how many layers she put on.

Her co-worker and close friend, Lisa, noticed her condition. "Sarah, you look awful. Are you sure you're okay?"

Sarah forced a weak smile. "I'm just feeling a bit under the weather. I'm planning to see the doctor after work."

Lisa looked concerned. "Don't wait. Go now. I'll cover for you."

Sarah hesitated but knew Lisa was right. "Thanks, Lisa. I'll head out now."

As Sarah drove to the doctor's office, her mind raced with thoughts. She tried to stay calm, convincing herself it was just a bad case of the flu. But deep down, she knew something was seriously wrong. Her heart pounded in her chest, and she had to grip the steering wheel tightly to keep her hands steady.

Even though it was only a short journey, the doctor's office seemed to take forever. Every turn felt more acute, every red light appeared to last longer. Her illness had worsened by the time she got there. She staggered toward the front desk area, her eyesight a little fuzzy.

Upon observing her condition, the receptionist promptly requested a nurse. After being led into an examination room, Sarah sat down still and began to breathe shallowly.

Entering the room was Dr. Williams, a seasoned doctor who had followed Sarah through her two pregnancies. His kind grin soon gave way to a worried expression as he observed her looks. "You don't look well at all, Sarah. Let's have you examined.

Her fever was startlingly high when he took it, and he also saw that her blood pressure was low and her pulse was quick. Sarah explained her symptoms to him while he examined her, including the fever, chills, aches in her muscles, and extreme exhaustion.

Dr. Williams scowled. These can indicate a serious infection. We must conduct some testing right now. In order to help stabilize Sarah's health, blood samples were collected and fluids were administered. Although they would have to wait for the test results, Dr. Williams said they suspected a significant bacterial infection. He advised her to return home, take it easy, and visit the ER if things got worse.

After the fluids, Sarah felt a little better but was still not feeling well when she got home. James had picked up the kids and was preparing dinner. He rushed to her side as she walked through the door. "How did it go?"

"They took some tests. Dr. Williams thinks it might be a severe infection. I just need to rest and wait for the results," she said, trying to sound reassuring.

James fetched her a blanket and assisted her to the couch. Sarah's condition worsened over the course of the evening. Her breathing became difficult, her fever increased, and she became more and more disoriented. James called Dr. Williams to give him an update on her condition, now overcome with panic.

"James, you need to take her to the emergency room immediately," Dr. Williams instructed. "This sounds like it could be septic shock. She needs urgent medical attention."

James acted without thinking. Sarah was taken into his arms and brought to the car by him. James's memory of the trip to the hospital was a haze of sirens and red lights, even though they hadn't requested an ambulance. He continued looking at Sarah, whose pale, clammy skin was sliding in and out of consciousness.

A group of medical experts greeted them at the hospital and promptly evaluated Sarah's health. After being taken to the emergency room, she was surrounded by a frenzy of activity from the nurses and physicians. As they attempted to steady her, James looked on helplessly. Snatches of medical terminology may be heard: "Blood pressure falling... Administer IV fluids first. Give antibiotics... Get ready to get intubated.

A doctor appeared out of the pandemonium and walked over to James. "Your wife is in septic shock, Mr. Peterson. We're making every effort to keep her stable. We must move swiftly to combat the illness and protect her essential organs. Sarah continued to be in critical condition as the night went on.

After being transferred to the intensive care unit (ICU), she was given a ventilator to aid with her breathing. In addition to drugs to keep her blood pressure stable, strong antibiotics were used to treat the illness.

Despite her unconsciousness, James remained by her side, holding her hand and conversing with her. The medical team put in a lot of overtime, keeping an eye on her vitals and modifying her therapy as necessary. There was a lot of uncertainty and worry during this stressful and terrible period. James and their family could barely remember the following few days. Sarah stayed in the intensive care unit, experiencing periods of stability and crises in her health. While the physicians exerted all of their might to combat the illness, they had to wait and watch how her body would react.

Friends and relatives helped James and the children during their days in the hospital by bringing food, praying for them, and taking turns sitting with them. James spent much of his time with Sarah, chatting to her, reading her books, and playing her favorite music in the hopes that she might hear him.

There was a ray of hope after a few days. Sarah's blood pressure normalized and her fever started to go down. The drugs seemed to be having an effect on the infection. After reducing the ventilator assistance progressively, Sarah's breathing became independent once more.

James experienced a wave of relief, but he also realized that recuperation would take time and effort. While the immediate crisis was passed, Sarah's journey had only begun. Sarah's condition quickly worsened while she lay in the emergency hospital.

Her fever, chills, and exhaustion had developed into something much darker than that. Although the medical staff acted quickly, Sarah's body appeared to be shutting down despite their best efforts. Her breathing had become difficult, her blood pressure was still dropping, and the temperature that had dogged her earlier in the day had now dangerously high.

The attending physician, Dr. Thomas, identified the symptoms of septic shock, a serious and potentially fatal illness that develops when the body's reaction to an infection results in extensive inflammation and organ failure. In order to find the infection's origins and decide on the best course of action, he promptly ordered a series of tests. Complete blood counts (CBCs), imaging examinations, and blood cultures were carried out promptly, but the results would not come in right away.

By Wednesday morning's early hours, Sarah's condition had gotten worse. Her blood pressure remained dangerously low even after receiving intravenous fluids and broad-spectrum antibiotics. Her heart was thumping rapidly, finding it difficult to circulate blood throughout her body. Sarah needed more intensive care and closer observation, so Dr. Thomas determined it was time to transfer her to the intensive care unit (ICU).

Sarah was taken into the ICU, James trailing closely after. His heart ached from fear and helplessness as he grasped her hand. Quickly taking over, the ICU doctors put her on vasopressors to narrow her blood vessels and increase her blood pressure. To help her breathe, they also started her on mechanical ventilation.

Sarah stood in the ICU, surrounded by a maze of tubes and equipment. The room was filled with the rhythmic hiss of the ventilator and the steady beep of the cardiac monitor. Doctors and nurses moved with well-honed precision, changing settings, giving her medication, and keeping an eye on her vitals. The ICU specialist,

Dr. Thomas, gave James an update on Sarah's health. "Your spouse is experiencing sepsis. While we battle the infection, we're doing everything we can to keep her body healthy. It's imperative to maintain a steady blood pressure and make sure her organs get enough oxygen.

In an attempt to process the seriousness of the situation, James nodded. He was torn between hope and dread, holding onto the hope that Sarah might survive.

Sarah's condition had not improved much by midmorning. Already strained, her kidneys started to fail. According to Dr. Thomas, this is a typical side effect of septic shock as the kidneys are extremely sensitive to variations in oxygenation and blood flow. Sarah's failing kidneys were supported by continuous renal replacement therapy (CRRT), a kind of dialysis intended for patients in critical condition. Elevated liver enzymes in her blood tests suggested a deterioration in her liver function.

To stop additional harm, the ICU staff continuously monitored her liver and gave supportive care.

James and their family's emotional toll increased as the day went on. Liam and Sophie, the children, were with their grandparents, who made an effort to keep things normal while protecting them from the worst of the news. Family members and friends paid the hospital a visit, bringing prayers and support. James stayed by Sarah's side for as long as he could. In an attempt to break through the fog of anesthesia and sickness, he conversed with her, read her favorite novels, and played recordings of their kids' voices.

Several times he found himself in the hospital chapel, looking for strength and comfort. He was troubled by the uncertainties surrounding Sarah's health, but he remained optimistic.

There was a slight but noticeable difference by sunset. Despite the vasopressors, Sarah's blood pressure, which had been dangerously low, started to stabilize. Carefully adjusting her medicine, Dr. Thomas and the ICU team hoped that her body was beginning to respond.

Even while Sarah's fever was still high, it was becoming lower. It appeared as though the drugs were gradually eliminating the infection that had destroyed her body. Her white blood cell count had somewhat improved, according to blood tests, indicating that her immune system was responding. James held fast to these rays of optimism. Though he was aware that they were still very much in the woods, any progress in this never-ending struggle was a success.

The ICU staff continued to provide attentive care as night fell. Sarah stayed on the ventilator, relying on the machine's constant beat to support her breathing. Although she still had impaired kidney function, the CRRT was assisting her in maintaining her fluid balance and eliminating toxins from her blood.

James and Dr. Thomas met to talk about the future strategy. "Sarah is still in critical condition, but there are encouraging indicators. It's critical that you keep a careful eye on her and modify her treatment as necessary. The crucial hours will be the following 24 to 48. James nodded, determination and tiredness mixed together in his eyes.

"I'm grateful, Dr. Thomas. I only want her to be alright. An nervous wait mixed with medical treatments made for a long night in the intensive care unit.
Seated in a chair by Sarah's bed, James slept fitfully, waking at every shift in the beeping monitors or the subdued chatter of the nurses.

He reflected on their lives together, their first college date, their wedding, Liam and Sophie's births. He reminisced about their many happy and loving occasions as well as their future goals. He could not stand to consider losing Sarah. The concept was agonizing. On Wednesday morning, the ICU team assembled for their shift change as daylight broke. Dr. Thomas gave the new team an update on Sarah's health and her overnight development. The understanding that septic shock was erratic and could change at any time created a cautious hope in the room.

Sarah's test results showed some slight improvements, and her vital signs were more stable. Her body was reacting to the harsh treatment, although a little slowly. In order to determine whether there are any bacteria still in her circulation and to modify her antibiotic regimen accordingly, Dr. Thomas ordered fresh blood cultures. The following few days were a waiting game interspersed with disappointments and hopeful moments. Sarah stayed in the ICU under the watchful eye of the medical staff and amid the incessant hum of machinery. James and their family kept a watch, their whole existence centered around her recuperation.

Little triumphs brought James comfort: Sarah's fever subsided, her renal function improved, and her blood pressure stabilized. Even if the road to recovery was still lengthy and unpredictable, every improvement was a step in the right direction.

Dr. Thomas gave the order, "Let's start an IV and get a full set of vitals." Blood cultures, CBC, lactate levels, and a full metabolic panel are required. Administer intravenous fluids and initiate broad-spectrum antibiotics for her. We must have her stabilized as soon as possible. The action in the room was humming.

Sarah's blood pressure was dangerously low when a nurse wrapped a blood pressure cuff on her arm. She started to receive much-needed hydration when a different nurse placed an IV line into her hand and started to drip fluids. Blood was drawn and sent to the lab for urgent analysis.

Sarah's skin looked pale and clammy, and her breathing was shallow and fast. Hearing her heart and lungs, Dr. Thomas observed her fast beating and short breathing. In an attempt to raise her oxygen levels, he adjusted the oxygen mask covering her face.

Dr. Thomas talked to James, who was standing close by, pale and nervous, while the team sought to stabilize Sarah. "Your spouse's condition is grave. We believe we have septic shock, a serious infection-related reaction. Her vital organs are not getting enough blood or oxygen, and her blood pressure is extremely low. We're exerting every effort to stabilize her and locate the infection's source.

James nodded, his mind racing. "What caused this? How did it get so bad so quickly?"

Dr. Thomas shook his head. "Septic shock can develop rapidly. Even a seemingly minor infection can trigger it if the body's immune response goes into overdrive. We'll know more once we get the lab results."

Dr. Thomas was right when the rapid lab results confirmed his concerns. Sarah had a very high white blood cell count, which suggested a serious infection. Her high lactate levels indicated that her body was not getting enough oxygen to the tissues. Blood samples confirmed the existence of a bacterial infection, but the precise strain would not be known for several days.

The parents of James and Sarah arrived at the hospital, and Dr. Thomas gave them an explanation of the situation. Sarah is experiencing widespread inflammation and organ malfunction as a result of her body's reaction to the infection, a condition known as septic shock. She is receiving fluids and antibiotics, but in order to receive more intensive treatment and close observation, she will need to be admitted to the intensive care unit.

James felt a wave of fear and helplessness wash over him. "What are her chances?"

Dr. Thomas met his gaze with a mixture of empathy and determination. "Septic shock is very serious, but we caught it early, and she's in good hands. We'll do everything we can to help her recover."

Sarah was sent to the Intensive Care Unit (ICU), where she was met by a highly skilled group of medical professionals. The ICU was a cold, artificial space where machines hummed and monitors beeped softly. Sarah was given a bed with gadgets all around it to track her vital signs and assist her failing organs.

Sarah's treatment was taken over by the ICU specialist, Dr. Thomas. She rapidly came up with a plan of action after going over the ER notes and the preliminary test results. Sarah's illness necessitated rigorous care and ongoing observation. Dr. Thomas gave her staff the order, "We'll continue the IV fluids and the broad-spectrum antibiotics." "Install vasopressors to keep her blood pressure stable and get ready for mechanical ventilation in case her breathing gets worse." We must continue to be ahead of this.

Sarah's body endured an unrelenting assault of medical procedures in the intensive care unit. In order to guarantee that blood and oxygen reached her essential organs, the vasopressors worked to narrow her blood arteries and increase her blood pressure. To enable regular blood drawing and to provide continuous blood pressure monitoring, an arterial line was placed.

Since Sarah's breathing continued to be difficult, Dr. Thomas decided to put her under an intubation. After a quick and accurate procedure, Sarah was quickly hooked up to a ventilator, which did her breathing for her. A reminder of the delicate balance being maintained was provided by the machine's constant rhythm, which filled the room.

Sarah's parents alternated between sitting by her bedside, their expressions filled with weariness and concern. Liam and Sophie, the kids, felt the anxiety and tension in the air even though they were too young to fully comprehend the seriousness of the situation. As best they could, Sarah's parents made an effort to keep them busy while offering consolation and confidence.

In an attempt to make his presence known to Sarah despite the sedation and machines, James spent as much time as he could chatting to her and holding her hand. He brought in family pictures and arranged them all over the space as a memento of the life they had together and the future they wanted to take back.

The next few days were a grueling test of endurance and resilience. Sarah's condition remained critical, but there were small signs of improvement. Her blood pressure began to stabilize, and her fever gradually subsided. The antibiotics were slowly taking effect, combating the bacterial infection that had ravaged her body.

Sarah was constantly observed by Dr. Thomas and her team, who made necessary adjustments to her medication and treatment regimen. They rejoiced at every tiny accomplishment, such as a decrease in fever, a minor enhancement in renal function, or a decrease in the requirement for vasopressors. Every improvement represented a step closer to recovery, but the road remained difficult and uncertain. James and his family held onto optimism and perseverance through it all. They found support in one another, in their friends and neighborhood, and in the committed medical staff who gave their all to preserve Sarah's life. They faced several obstacles on the way, but they didn't give up.

Chapter Two

The Fight for Life : Intensive care in the intensive care unit

Sarah's rapidly deteriorating condition required an urgent transfer to the intensive care unit. The ICU was an other universe, a sterile, bleak space where cutting-edge medical equipment hummed. The doctors and nurses moved with a trained precision, the weight of their obligations and their physical coverings hiding their features. The air was filled with the quiet murmur of medical workers, the hiss of ventilators, and the beeping of monitors.

Sarah was hooked up right away to a number of devices that would continuously check her vital signs. Her wrist was fitted with an arterial line to monitor her blood pressure continuously and enable regular blood draws without the need for further needle sticks. In order to monitor her heart rate and rhythm, a cardiac monitor was connected to her, and a pulse oximeter was fastened to her finger to gauge the blood's oxygen saturation.

At the heart of this chaos was the ICU specialist, Dr. Thomas, who was commanding her team with cool composure. Upon reviewing Sarah's chart, she observed that IV fluids and broad-spectrum antibiotics had previously been given in the emergency room. Her greatest worry at this point was Sarah's blood pressure, which was dangerously low even after the first interventions. Vasopressors are strong drugs that constrict blood arteries and elevate blood pressure. Dr. Thomas ordered their administration. In order to guarantee that Sarah's key organs received adequate blood flow, this was an essential step. Sarah's huge neck vein was punctured by the ICU nurse to create a central line, which gave the vasopressors and other drugs a direct path to her body.

"Start her on norepinephrine," Dr. Thomas instructed. "We need to get her MAP (mean arterial pressure) above 65."

With a quick adjustment of the infusion pump, the drug started to enter Sarah's system. Her blood pressure started to rise in a matter of minutes, but it stayed unstable. Dr. Thomas kept a careful eye on the readings and was prepared to change the dosage as necessary. Another big worry was Sarah's respiration. She was breathing quickly and had dangerously low oxygen levels. It was decided to intubate her and put her on a mechanical ventilator, which would act as her personal breathing apparatus.

The intubation process was carried out expertly. To make sure Sarah was unconscious and not in pain, a sedative was given to her. With caution, a tube was placed through her mouth and into her trachea before being attached to the ventilator. The machine started to give her controlled breaths, making sure her lungs got enough oxygen and were able to release carbon dioxide effectively.

It became clear over the next few hours that Sarah's kidneys weren't working correctly. Her blood tests revealed increasing levels of creatinine and other waste products, and she produced very little urine. Because there is less blood supply to the kidneys in septic shock, acute renal damage is a typical consequence that Dr. Thomas identified.

Sarah was put on continuous renal replacement treatment (CRRT), a kind of dialysis intended for patients in critical condition, to support her kidneys. After inserting a catheter into a sizable vein, the CRRT machine started to continually filter her blood, eliminating waste materials and surplus fluids while preserving the proper balance of electrolytes.

Maintaining Sarah's nutritional health was another problem, as she was sedated and unable to eat. A nasogastric (NG) tube—a thin, flexible tube that went through her nose and into her stomach—was implanted by the ICU team. With the use of this tube, liquid nutrition may be given to her, supporting her body's recovery process with vital nutrients including vitamins, proteins, and calories.

Sarah's status was continuously checked in the intensive care unit. Every hour, nurses would check her vital signs, and daily lab tests would be conducted to monitor her progress. To assess Sarah's condition and modify her treatment plan as necessary, Dr. Thomas and her team met on a frequent basis.

The antibiotics were tailored based on the results of the blood cultures, which identified the specific bacteria causing the infection. Additional medications were given to manage pain, control her fever, and prevent complications like blood clots and gastrointestinal bleeding.

Sarah's family endured an emotional rollercoaster as she battled for her life in the intensive care unit. Even though she was profoundly unconscious and did not know he was there, James stayed by her side for as long as he could, holding her hand and talking to her. He brought pictures of their kids, Liam and Sophie, and arranged them all over the space to serve as a memento of the life they had created.

Robert and Helen, Sarah's parents, provided unwavering support. They alternated in sitting with Sarah, bringing encouraging words and prayers. Frequently, Helen would caress Sarah's hair, murmuring tales from her early years and reassuring her of the love and encouragement that awaited her at home.

Liam and Sophie's grandparents kept them busy because they were too little to realize how serious the situation was. When they could, they went to see Sarah. They brought her pictures and spoke about their school days. Their harmless banter provided a tiny but essential bit of normalcy in a world gone crazy. Sarah's condition persisted in being critical even after receiving intense care. Although the vasopressors assisted in bringing her blood pressure under control, her body was still battling a serious infection. Although the bacterium was killed by the medications, the inflammatory response still caused havoc with her organs.

Dr. Thomas and her colleagues continued to monitor Sarah closely and frequently modified her course of therapy. They kept an eye out for indications that she was getting better, such more urine production, blood pressure stability without the need for vasopressors, and a decrease in inflammatory markers in her blood tests. Little but meaningful improvements were seen after many days in the intensive care unit. Sarah's white blood cell count returned to normal and her fever started to drop, suggesting that the infection was starting to get under control.

Early indicators of renal function improvement were a progressive rise in urine production. These modest triumphs gave Sarah's family and the medical staff a ray of optimism. Dr. Thomas cautioned that Sarah's recovery would be a long and difficult journey, but the initial progress was a positive sign.

As Sarah's health gradually improved, attention turned to her long-term recuperation. In order to rebuild her strength and recuperate from the psychological and physical effects of septic shock, she would require prolonged therapy. Her ultimate transfer to a step-down facility, where she would continue her recuperation under close medical observation, was being planned by the ICU team.

James and his family did not waver in their support of one another, finding solace in one another and the committed medical staff. They were committed to helping Sarah regain her life even though they understood the journey ahead would be difficult.

Following a number of tough days in the intensive care unit, Sarah's health started to recover. Her vital signs and lab findings changed little but significantly at this point, indicating that the harsh therapies were beginning to have an impact. Sarah's fever gradually decreased, which was one of the first indications that she was getting well. Her body's constant high temperatures started to drop, indicating that the antibiotics were successfully treating the infection. Her body, stuck in a vicious cycle of chills and sweats brought on by fever, began to regulate its temperature somewhat.

With cautious optimism, Dr. Thomas noted Sarah's fever had decreased. "This is encouraging," she said to James. In other words, the antibiotics are effective. Though it's not yet clear cut, this is a move in the right direction.

Sarah's blood pressure started to stabilize after being dangerously low despite receiving vasopressors continuously. Sarah's body was able to do more work as the ICU team gradually lowered the dosage of these medications. Every decrease in vasopressors was a fine balance that was closely watched to make sure her blood pressure didn't go over a safe limit.

Sarah's circulatory system shown resiliency as the vasopressors were reduced. Her organs were getting enough blood and oxygen, as seen by the stable mean arterial pressure (MAP) reading. Her recovery reached a critical turning point with this stabilization. Sarah's respiratory condition was also getting better. Her lungs were given more freedom to breathe by progressively adjusting the mechanical ventilator that had been supporting her breathing. Weaning entailed gradually lowering the ventilator's assistance while keeping an eye on Sarah's capacity to breathe on her own.

Sarah's breathing patterns, oxygen saturation, and carbon dioxide levels were continuously monitored by the respiratory therapists and intensive care unit nurses. They became increasingly optimistic that she would soon be able to breathe on her own with every tweak that went well. The increase in Sarah's urine output was one of the most positive indicators of recovery. After being seriously damaged by the septic shock, her kidneys started to recover. Her kidneys were supported during this crucial time by continuous renal replacement treatment (CRRT), which allowed them to gradually start functioning again.

As Sarah's blood waste products and creatinine levels decreased, Dr. Thomas kept an eye on her lab findings. These modifications meant that she wouldn't require as much intense dialysis because her kidneys were beginning to remove toxins more efficiently. Further indications of stabilization were found by Sarah's blood tests. As the infection subsided, her white blood cell count, which had been dangerously elevated, started to return to normal. Procalcitonin and C-reactive protein (CRP) levels, two inflammatory markers that indicate a decline in systemic inflammation, also trended downward.

The fact that these lab results returned to normal demonstrated the body's capacity to recuperate from serious sickness given the appropriate care. Dr. Thomas and her group kept a careful eye on these indicators and modified Sarah's treatment approach as necessary. The ICU staff started the process of weaning Sarah off the sedatives that had kept her calm and unconscious during the most dangerous parts of her illness as her condition got better. In order to prevent withdrawal symptoms and guarantee Sarah's comfort, this process needs to be carefully monitored. The sedative infusions were tapered off gradually, and Sarah began to regain her composure. She started to respond to basic commands, move her fingers, and open her eyes. These small movements were met with joy and relief by her family, who had been anxiously waiting for any sign of awareness.

As Sarah's sedation was decreased, she became more aware of her surroundings and began to interact with her family. James, who had been by her side throughout the ordeal, held her hand and spoke to her softly. Sarah's eyes, once clouded by sedation and illness, began to show recognition and emotion.

The first time Sarah squeezed James's hand in response was a moment of profound relief and hope. Tears welled in his eyes as he realized that Sarah was beginning to emerge from the depths of her critical illness.

Sarah's parents, Helen and Robert, were also present during these early moments of reconnection. Helen spoke to Sarah, recounting fond memories and expressing her love and support. Robert, usually a stoic figure, could not hide his emotions as he watched his daughter slowly return to consciousness.

With Sarah's increasing responsiveness, the ICU team introduced physical therapy to prevent muscle atrophy and improve her overall strength. The physical therapists started with passive range-of-motion exercises, gently moving Sarah's limbs to maintain flexibility and circulation.

As Sarah regained more strength, she was encouraged to sit up in bed with assistance. This was a significant step, as prolonged bed rest and immobility could lead to muscle weakness and complications like blood clots and pressure ulcers.

Sarah's physical therapists and nurses supported her during these early mobilization efforts, celebrating each small achievement. Sitting up for a few minutes, moving her legs, and eventually standing with support were milestones in her journey toward recovery.

Throughout Sarah's stabilization process, the dedication and expertise of the ICU team were unwavering. Dr. Thomas and her colleagues held regular multidisciplinary meetings to discuss Sarah's progress and adjust her treatment plan as needed. They remained vigilant for any signs of setbacks, ready to intervene at the slightest hint of trouble.

The ICU nurses, respiratory therapists, and other staff members provided continuous care and support, ensuring that Sarah's needs were met around the clock. Their compassion and professionalism were instrumental in her recovery.

The emotional toll of Sarah's illness extended beyond her immediate family to include the healthcare providers who cared for her. Recognizing the psychological impact of critical illness on both patients and their families, the ICU offered counseling and support services.

James and Sarah's parents availed themselves of these resources, finding solace in talking to therapists and support groups who understood the unique challenges they faced. Sharing their fears, hopes, and experiences with others who had walked similar paths provided a sense of community and strength.

As Sarah's condition continued to stabilize, the ICU team began to prepare for her transfer to a step-down unit, where she would receive ongoing care while gradually transitioning to less intensive medical support. This next phase of her recovery would focus on regaining strength, mobility, and independence.

The transfer to the step-down unit was a significant milestone, marking the end of the most critical phase of Sarah's illness. While the road to full recovery remained long and challenging, the signs of improvement and stabilization were a testament to the resilience of the human body and spirit.

After days of intensive care and monitoring, Sarah's condition had stabilized significantly. The ICU team, led by Dr.

Thomas, assessed her progress daily, carefully weighing the decision to transfer her to a less intensive setting. This decision was not made lightly, as it marked a pivotal step in Sarah's recovery journey.

Dr. Thomas gathered her team for a detailed discussion on Sarah's status. "Sarah's vitals have stabilized, her infection is under control, and she's showing consistent signs of improvement," she began. "I believe it's time to consider transferring her to a regular ward where she can continue her recovery with less intensive monitoring."

The team agreed, noting Sarah's improved blood pressure, respiratory function, and kidney performance. She was now off vasopressors, her breathing was supported only by supplemental oxygen, and her kidneys were functioning well enough to discontinue dialysis. These improvements indicated that she no longer required the constant, high-level care of the ICU.

Preparing for Transfer

The preparation for Sarah's transfer was meticulous. The ICU nurses compiled a detailed report of her current condition, medications, and treatment protocols to ensure a smooth transition. Dr. Thomas personally briefed Dr. Anne Carter, the physician who would oversee Sarah's care in the regular ward.

"Sarah still needs close monitoring for any signs of relapse or complications," Dr. Thomas emphasized. "Her recovery is progressing well, but we need to ensure continuity in her care plan."

Dr. Carter nodded, understanding the gravity of the responsibility. "We'll make sure she continues to receive the best care. Our team is ready for her."

For Sarah's family, the news of her transfer was a mix of relief and anxiety. James, who had been by her side throughout the ordeal, was both hopeful and cautious. "It's a good sign that she's moving out of the ICU, right?" he asked Dr. Thomas, seeking reassurance.

"Yes, it is," Dr. Thomas replied with a reassuring smile. "It means she's making significant progress. But remember, the recovery process is ongoing. She'll still need support and care."

Helen and Robert, Sarah's parents, were relieved to hear that their daughter was improving enough to leave the ICU. Helen hugged James tightly, tears of relief streaming down her face. "She's coming back to us," she whispered.

The Transfer Process

On the day of the transfer, the ICU team worked efficiently to ensure everything was in place. Sarah's medications were carefully packed, her IV lines were checked, and her medical records were updated. The transport team arrived with a stretcher, ready to move her to the regular ward.

James and the family watched anxiously as Sarah was gently transferred to the stretcher. Although still weak and drowsy, Sarah managed a faint smile when she saw her family gathered around. It was a moment of hope, a sign that she was slowly coming back to them.

The regular ward was a quieter environment compared to the bustling ICU. Sarah was wheeled into a private room, where the atmosphere was less clinical and more conducive to rest and recovery. Dr. Carter and her team were there to welcome Sarah and ensure she was settled comfortably.

"We're glad to have you here, Sarah," Dr. Carter said warmly. "You're in good hands, and we'll do everything we can to support your continued recovery."

The nurses in the regular ward were briefed on Sarah's condition and care plan. They took over the monitoring of her vital signs, administered her medications, and provided the necessary support to aid her recovery.

For Sarah, the transition to the regular ward was both a relief and an adjustment. The constant beeping of ICU monitors was replaced by a more peaceful silence, but she also felt the absence of the continuous attention she had grown accustomed to. It was a step towards independence, but it also required her to adapt to a new level of self-reliance.

James and the family spent as much time as possible with Sarah, helping her adjust to the new environment. They brought familiar items from home—her favorite blanket, photos, and books—to make her room feel more like a sanctuary. Their presence provided comfort and motivation, reminding Sarah of the life she was fighting to reclaim.

In the regular ward, Sarah's care plan continued to be comprehensive. She was still on a course of antibiotics to ensure the infection was fully eradicated. Her nutritional needs were met through a carefully planned diet, and physical therapy sessions were scheduled to help her regain strength and mobility.

The regular monitoring of Sarah's vital signs remained crucial. Nurses checked her temperature, blood pressure, heart rate, and oxygen levels regularly, looking for any signs of complications or setbacks. Blood tests were conducted to monitor her kidney function, electrolyte balance, and overall health status.

Physical therapy played a vital role in Sarah's recovery. The therapists designed a personalized exercise program to help her regain strength and mobility gradually. Initially, the focus was on passive range-of-motion exercises to prevent muscle atrophy and maintain joint flexibility.

As Sarah's strength improved, the therapy sessions became more active. She was encouraged to sit up in bed, move her legs, and eventually stand with support. Each small achievement was a step towards regaining her independence.

"Take it slow, Sarah," the physical therapist advised during one session. "You're doing great. Remember, it's all about gradual progress."

Sarah's determination was evident. Despite the fatigue and occasional pain, she pushed herself to participate actively in the therapy sessions. The support and encouragement from her family and the medical team fueled her motivation to recover.

The psychological impact of Sarah's ordeal could not be overlooked. The trauma of septic shock and the prolonged ICU stay had left emotional scars that needed healing. The hospital's support services included counseling for Sarah and her family to help them navigate the emotional challenges of recovery.

Sarah's sessions with the counselor provided a safe space to express her fears, frustrations, and hopes. She talked about the anxiety of her sudden illness, the helplessness she felt during her ICU stay, and her determination to regain her life.

"Your feelings are completely valid, Sarah," the counselor reassured her. "Recovery isn't just about the physical aspects. It's also about healing emotionally and finding your inner strength."

James also found solace in these counseling sessions. Sharing his fears and experiences with someone who understood the psychological toll of such a traumatic event helped him cope with the emotional strain. The sessions provided him with tools to support Sarah's emotional recovery while taking care of his own mental health.

As the days passed, Sarah began to establish a new routine in the regular ward. She woke up to the comforting presence of her family, engaged in physical therapy sessions, and participated in counseling. Her strength gradually returned, and she became more involved in her care.

The nursing staff supported Sarah's efforts to regain independence. They encouraged her to perform basic self-care tasks, such as brushing her teeth and washing her face.

These small activities were milestones in her journey towards regaining autonomy.

Each milestone in Sarah's recovery was celebrated with joy and relief. The first time she walked a few steps with the help of a walker was a moment of triumph. James and the family cheered her on, their hearts filled with pride and hope.

"You're amazing, Sarah," James said, tears of happiness in his eyes. "You're getting stronger every day."

These celebrations, though small in the grand scheme of recovery, were vital in maintaining Sarah's motivation and morale. They reminded her of the progress she was making and the love and support surrounding her.

As Sarah continued to improve, the medical team began to discuss the possibility of her discharge from the hospital. Dr. Carter and the nurses worked closely with Sarah and her family to prepare for this transition. It was essential to ensure that Sarah would receive the necessary care and support at home.

A comprehensive discharge plan was developed, outlining the medications Sarah needed to continue, follow-up appointments with her healthcare providers, and the continuation of physical therapy. The family was also educated on recognizing potential signs of complications and when to seek medical attention.

Chapter Three

Transition from critical condition to gradual recovery

After the critical days spent in the ICU, Sarah's condition began to show promising signs of improvement and stabilization. This phase was marked by a series of small yet significant victories that brought hope to her family and the medical team. Each indicator of progress was a testament to the efficacy of the treatment and Sarah's resilience.

One of the earliest signs of improvement was the regulation of Sarah's body temperature. Initially, her fever had been dangerously high, a clear indication of the severe infection raging within her body. As the antibiotics took effect, Sarah's fever began to subside. Her temperature stabilized, which was a crucial indicator that the infection was being brought under control.

Dr. Thomas, observing the consistent drop in Sarah's fever, felt a cautious optimism. "Sarah's body is responding well to the antibiotics," she explained to James. "This is a very positive sign."

Stabilizing Blood Pressure

Sarah's blood pressure had been a critical concern from the outset, necessitating the use of vasopressors to maintain adequate levels. As her condition improved, the medical team was able to gradually reduce the dosage of these medications. Each reduction was carefully monitored to ensure that Sarah's blood pressure remained stable without the need for continuous pharmaceutical support.

The stabilization of her blood pressure meant that her cardiovascular system was beginning to function more autonomously. This was a significant milestone, as it indicated that her body was starting to recover from the shock.

Another vital sign of improvement was in Sarah's respiratory function. The mechanical ventilator that had been supporting her breathing was gradually adjusted to allow her lungs to take over more of the work. This weaning process involved careful reduction in the ventilator settings and close monitoring of Sarah's ability to maintain adequate oxygen levels independently.

The respiratory therapists worked with Sarah, encouraging her to breathe deeply and steadily. Over time, her lung function improved, and she required less mechanical support. This progress was a hopeful sign that her respiratory system was healing.
Sarah's kidneys, which had been severely affected by the septic shock, also began to show signs of recovery. Her urine output increased, indicating that her kidneys were starting to function more effectively. The continuous renal replacement therapy (CRRT) that had supported her during the critical phase was gradually tapered off as her kidneys resumed their role in filtering waste from her blood.

Dr. Thomas monitored the lab results closely, noting the declining levels of creatinine and other waste products in Sarah's blood. These improvements in kidney function were crucial, as they reduced the risk of further complications and supported her overall recovery.

Blood tests provided a detailed picture of Sarah's internal recovery. Her white blood cell count, which had been elevated due to the infection, began to normalize. Inflammatory markers such as C-reactive protein (CRP) and procalcitonin levels also showed a steady decline, indicating a reduction in systemic inflammation.

These lab results were closely watched by the medical team. The normalization of these values was a clear indicator that Sarah's body was overcoming the infection and the inflammatory response was subsiding.

As Sarah's physical condition improved, the need for heavy sedation decreased. The medical team began the delicate process of weaning her off sedative medications. This process was handled carefully to avoid withdrawal symptoms and ensure Sarah's comfort.

Gradually, Sarah became more aware and responsive. She started to open her eyes and respond to simple commands. Her first coherent words, although faint and labored, were a moment of profound joy for her family. These small signs of consciousness were a testament to her body's resilience and a beacon of hope for her loved ones.

With the decrease in sedation, Sarah was able to reconnect with her family. James, who had been by her side throughout, was the first to see the flicker of recognition in her eyes. He held her hand and spoke softly to her, sharing updates about their children and recounting memories. Sarah's faint smile and gentle squeeze of his hand were powerful affirmations of her improving condition.

Helen and Robert, Sarah's parents, also spent time with her, sharing stories and expressing their love. Their emotional support played a crucial role in Sarah's psychological recovery, providing her with the strength and motivation to keep fighting.

Physical therapy was introduced as soon as Sarah was stable enough. The therapists started with passive range-of-motion exercises to prevent muscle atrophy and maintain joint flexibility. As Sarah regained strength, the sessions progressed to more active exercises.

Sarah's determination was evident as she engaged in these sessions, despite the fatigue and discomfort. With the support of the physical therapists, she began to sit up, move her limbs, and eventually stand with assistance. These small steps were significant milestones in her journey towards regaining mobility and independence.

The psychological impact of Sarah's ordeal was substantial. Recognizing this, the hospital provided counseling services to support her emotional recovery. Sarah's sessions with the counselor allowed her to express her fears and frustrations, and to begin processing the trauma she had experienced.

James also participated in counseling, finding it helpful to share his own fears and hopes. The emotional support they received was crucial in helping them cope with the challenges of recovery and maintain their mental well-being.

As Sarah's physical condition stabilized, the focus shifted to building her strength and endurance. Nutritional support played a vital role in this phase. A carefully planned diet ensured she received the necessary calories, proteins, and vitamins to aid her body's healing process.

Sarah's daily routine included nutritious meals, physical therapy, and periods of rest. Each day brought small but significant improvements. Her ability to perform basic self-care tasks, such as brushing her teeth and washing her face, marked important steps towards independence.

Throughout this period, Sarah's family remained her strongest support system. James and the children visited regularly, bringing drawings, letters, and stories from home. These visits lifted Sarah's spirits and provided her with a sense of normalcy and connection to the life she was striving to return to.

Helen and Robert took turns staying with Sarah, offering emotional support and encouragement. Their presence provided a sense of security and comfort, reinforcing Sarah's determination to recover.

Each milestone in Sarah's recovery was celebrated with joy and gratitude. The first time she stood on her own, the first steps she took with a walker, and the day she no longer needed supplemental oxygen were all moments of triumph. These achievements were shared with her family and the medical team, who had been instrumental in her journey.

As Sarah's condition continued to improve, discussions began about her transfer from the ICU to a regular ward. This move was a significant step towards her eventual discharge from the hospital. The medical team prepared a comprehensive plan to ensure a smooth transition, focusing on maintaining the progress she had made and addressing any ongoing needs.

A Major Milestone

After enduring the intense battle in the ICU, Sarah's improving condition indicated she was ready for the next phase of her recovery. The decision to transfer her from the ICU to a regular ward was a significant milestone, symbolizing a crucial step towards her return to normalcy.

The ICU team, led by Dr. Thomas, held a series of discussions to evaluate Sarah's readiness for transfer. They meticulously reviewed her vitals, lab results, and overall stability. Sarah had shown consistent signs of improvement: her blood pressure was stable without the need for vasopressors, her breathing was no longer reliant on mechanical ventilation, and her kidney function was returning to normal.

Dr. Thomas addressed her colleagues, "Sarah's progress has been remarkable. Her vitals have stabilized, and her infection is under control. I believe she's ready to transition to the regular ward, where she can continue her recovery with less intensive monitoring."

The team concurred, understanding that this move was not only a medical decision but also a psychological boost for Sarah and her family.

James and Sarah's parents, Helen and Robert, were informed about the planned transfer. The news was met with a mix of relief and apprehension. They understood that moving out of the ICU meant Sarah was no longer in critical condition, but they also knew that her recovery journey was far from over.

"It's a good sign that Sarah is moving out of the ICU," Dr. Thomas reassured them. "This means she's making significant progress. The regular ward will allow her to continue her recovery in a less intense environment, but she will still receive all the care she needs."

James, holding Helen's hand, nodded. "We're grateful for the progress she's made. We'll be with her every step of the way."

The day of the transfer was carefully planned to ensure Sarah's comfort and safety. The ICU nurses prepared her medical records, medications, and necessary equipment for the move. Sarah was gently transferred to a stretcher, with James and her parents by her side, offering words of encouragement.

As she was wheeled through the hospital corridors, Sarah's eyes flickered with awareness, and she managed a faint smile. The sight of her family and the change in surroundings provided a welcome change and a sense of forward momentum.

Sarah's arrival at the regular ward marked a new chapter in her recovery. Her room was quieter and more private compared to the bustling ICU. It was designed to provide a peaceful environment conducive to healing. The medical team in the regular ward, led by Dr. Anne Carter, welcomed Sarah warmly.

"We're glad to have you here, Sarah," Dr. Carter said. "You've made incredible progress, and we'll continue to support you every step of the way."

The nurses in the regular ward received a comprehensive handover from the ICU team, ensuring a seamless transition in care. They were briefed on Sarah's condition, medications, and ongoing treatment plan.
The regular ward offered Sarah a more relaxed atmosphere, but the transition required adjustment. The constant, vigilant

monitoring of the ICU was replaced by periodic checks, which meant Sarah had more privacy but also needed to adapt to a new level of independence.

James and her parents helped Sarah settle into her new room. They brought familiar items from home—photos, her favorite blanket, and a few personal belongings—to make the space feel more comforting and homelike. Their presence provided immense emotional support, easing Sarah's adjustment to the new environment.

Although Sarah had moved to the regular ward, her medical care remained rigorous. She continued on a course of antibiotics to ensure the infection was completely eradicated. Her vital signs were monitored regularly, and blood tests were conducted to track her recovery progress.

Sarah's care plan also included physical therapy sessions to help her regain strength and mobility. The physical therapists designed exercises tailored to her condition, gradually increasing the intensity as she gained strength. The goal was to restore her physical function and prevent complications like muscle atrophy.

Sarah's physical therapy sessions were a critical component of her recovery. Initially, the focus was on passive exercises to maintain joint flexibility and prevent stiffness. As she gained strength, the exercises became more active, encouraging her to move her limbs and sit up in bed.

One of the most significant milestones was the day Sarah stood up with assistance. Her legs trembled with the effort, but the determination in her eyes was unmistakable. With each session, she grew stronger, taking small but steady steps towards regaining her mobility.

"You're doing great, Sarah," her physical therapist encouraged. "Each step, no matter how small, is a victory."

The emotional and psychological aspects of Sarah's recovery were just as important as the physical ones. The trauma of septic shock and the intensive care experience had left deep emotional scars. Sarah continued to receive counseling to help her process her feelings and build resilience.

James and her parents also benefited from counseling services. They shared their experiences, fears, and hopes, finding solace in the support offered by the hospital's psychological team. These sessions helped them stay strong for Sarah and provided them with coping strategies to deal with the ongoing stress.

In the regular ward, Sarah began to establish a new daily routine. Mornings started with vital checks and a nutritious breakfast tailored to her dietary needs. Physical therapy sessions followed, interspersed with periods of rest. The afternoons were reserved for visits from her family, who brought stories and updates from home, lifting her spirits.

The nurses encouraged Sarah to participate in self-care activities as much as possible. Tasks like brushing her teeth and combing her hair, though simple, were important steps towards regaining her independence and self-confidence.

The medical team in the regular ward remained vigilant for any signs of complications. Sarah's blood pressure, heart rate, and oxygen levels were closely monitored. Regular blood tests checked her kidney function and overall health status. Any deviations from the expected recovery path were addressed promptly to prevent setbacks.

Dr. Carter and her team held regular meetings to review Sarah's progress and adjust her treatment plan as needed. This multidisciplinary approach ensured that all aspects of her recovery were considered and addressed.

Every small achievement in Sarah's recovery was celebrated. The first time she walked a few steps unassisted, the day she no longer needed supplemental oxygen, and her ability to eat solid food were all significant milestones. These moments were shared with her family and the medical team, creating a sense of accomplishment and hope.

"You're making amazing progress, Sarah," Dr. Carter said during one of her rounds. "Your determination and strength are truly inspiring."

As Sarah's condition continued to improve, discussions about her eventual discharge from the hospital began. Dr. Carter and the nursing team worked closely with Sarah and her family to prepare for this transition. The goal was to ensure that Sarah would continue to receive the necessary care and support at home.

A detailed discharge plan was developed, outlining her medication regimen, follow-up appointments with healthcare providers, and the continuation of physical therapy. Sarah's family was educated on recognizing signs of potential complications and when to seek medical attention.

Chapter Four

Psychological impact of the experience

Sarah's battle with septic shock left not only physical scars but also profound psychological ones. The abruptness of her illness, the intense fight for survival, and the long road to recovery created a whirlwind of emotions. The psychological impact of her experience was multifaceted, affecting her mental health, her relationships, and her overall outlook on life.

The initial phase of Sarah's recovery was dominated by fear and anxiety. The memory of waking up in the ICU, surrounded by machines and unfamiliar faces, haunted her. The realization that she had been on the brink of death was overwhelming. These thoughts often led to anxiety attacks, triggered by medical procedures or even the sound of beeping monitors.

Sarah's fear was not just about her past ordeal but also about her future. She worried about potential complications, the possibility of recurrence, and her ability to return to her previous active lifestyle. This anxiety manifested in sleepless nights, a heightened sense of vulnerability, and an aversion to anything that reminded her of the hospital environment.

The trauma of experiencing septic shock and the subsequent ICU stay had a lasting impact on Sarah's mental health. She exhibited symptoms of post-traumatic stress disorder (PTSD), including flashbacks, nightmares, and hypervigilance. Certain triggers, such as the smell of antiseptic or the sight of medical equipment, could send her into a panic.

Counseling sessions with a trauma specialist became an integral part of Sarah's recovery. These sessions provided a safe space for her to articulate her fears and process the trauma. The therapist employed techniques such as cognitive-behavioral therapy (CBT) and eye movement desensitization and reprocessing (EMDR) to help Sarah manage her symptoms and gradually reduce their intensity.

Sarah's emotional state fluctuated dramatically during her recovery. There were moments of deep gratitude for having survived, followed by periods of intense sadness and frustration. She mourned the loss of her former life, the energy and independence she once had. These emotions were compounded by the physical limitations she now faced, making everyday tasks seem daunting.

James, her husband, and their children provided a steady source of support, but they too struggled to navigate the emotional rollercoaster. Family counseling sessions helped them understand the psychological impact of Sarah's experience and equipped them with tools to support her effectively. These sessions also provided a platform for open communication, allowing each family member to express their feelings and concerns.

Struggles with Identity

Before her illness, Sarah's identity was closely tied to her active lifestyle and her role as a mother and wife. The sudden shift from being a vibrant, energetic person to someone who needed assistance for basic tasks was a profound blow to her self-esteem. She grappled with feelings of inadequacy and a sense of loss of self.

Rebuilding her identity became a crucial aspect of Sarah's psychological recovery. With the help of her therapist, she began to explore new aspects of herself, finding strength in her resilience and determination. She started to engage in activities that she could manage, such as reading, writing, and even light physical exercises tailored to her condition. These activities helped her rediscover a sense of purpose and self-worth.

Survivor's guilt was another significant psychological challenge for Sarah. She often found herself questioning why she survived when many others did not. This guilt was exacerbated by news stories of people succumbing to sepsis and other severe infections. She felt a deep sense of empathy for these individuals and their families, which sometimes led to overwhelming feelings of sadness and helplessness.

Therapy sessions addressed these feelings by helping Sarah understand that her survival was not a matter of fairness or deservingness, but rather a combination of timely medical intervention, her body's response, and sheer luck. Gradually, Sarah learned to channel her empathy into positive actions, such as supporting awareness campaigns for sepsis and sharing her story to inspire others.

While Sarah's experience put a strain on her family relationships, it also created opportunities for deepening their bonds. The ordeal highlighted the importance of communication, mutual support, and understanding. James and the children learned to be patient and compassionate, recognizing the invisible battles Sarah was fighting.

Family therapy sessions were instrumental in this process. They provided a structured environment for each family member to express their emotions and learn coping strategies. Over time, these sessions strengthened their relationships, fostering a sense of unity and resilience.

As Sarah navigated her psychological recovery, she discovered a new sense of purpose. Her experience had given her a profound appreciation for life and a desire to make a difference. She began to engage in activities that aligned with this newfound purpose, such as volunteering at local health awareness events and participating in support groups for septic shock survivors.

Sarah also started writing about her journey, using her story to raise awareness about septic shock and the importance of timely medical intervention. This endeavor not only provided her with a therapeutic outlet but also allowed her to connect with others who had similar experiences.

The journey towards psychological healing was long and arduous, but gradually, Sarah began to find acceptance. She acknowledged the trauma she had endured and the changes it had brought to her life. With the support of her family, friends, and healthcare professionals, she learned to embrace her new reality and focus on the positives.

Sarah's acceptance was not about forgetting her ordeal but about integrating it into her life in a way that allowed her to move forward. She recognized her strength and resilience, celebrating the progress she had made and the challenges she had overcome.

Sarah's psychological recovery was not a linear process. There were setbacks and difficult days, but ongoing support from her therapist, family, and support groups played a crucial role in her continued healing. She remained committed to her counseling sessions and engaged in activities that nurtured her mental well-being.

Her family also continued to play a vital role in her recovery, providing love, understanding, and encouragement. They celebrated her milestones, no matter how small, and stood by her during the challenging moments.

Chapter Five

Adoption of a Healthier Lifestyle

Sarah's near-death experience with septic shock served as a powerful catalyst for change. As she transitioned from the hospital back to her everyday life, she was determined to embrace a healthier lifestyle that would support her recovery and overall well-being. This journey towards health and wellness became a crucial part of her new beginning.

The first step in Sarah's journey was to evaluate her previous lifestyle habits. Before her illness, Sarah had been active but not always mindful of her nutritional choices or stress levels. The demands of family life, work, and social commitments often left little time for self-care. Reflecting on these habits helped Sarah recognize areas that needed improvement.

She realized that while she had always been physically active, her diet was often inconsistent, and she didn't prioritize rest and mental well-being. This self-assessment provided a foundation for the changes she was about to make.

Building a Nutrient-Rich Diet

Sarah understood that proper nutrition was vital for her recovery and long-term health. She consulted a nutritionist who helped her develop a balanced, nutrient-rich diet. Together, they crafted a meal plan that included a variety of fruits, vegetables, lean proteins, whole grains, and healthy fats.

The nutritionist emphasized the importance of incorporating foods rich in antioxidants, vitamins, and minerals to boost Sarah's immune system and support healing. Sarah began to experiment with new recipes, discovering a love for cooking meals that were both delicious and nutritious. She made a conscious effort to include superfoods like berries, leafy greens, nuts, and seeds in her diet.

Hydration became a key focus for Sarah. She learned that proper hydration was essential for overall health and particularly important for her recovering body. Sarah started drinking more water throughout the day, setting reminders to ensure she stayed hydrated.

In addition to water, she incorporated herbal teas and infused waters into her routine. These beverages not only kept her hydrated but also provided additional nutrients and antioxidants. Sarah noticed that staying well-hydrated improved her energy levels, digestion, and overall sense of well-being.

Regular Physical Activity

Although Sarah had always been active, she now approached physical activity with a renewed sense of purpose. Her physical therapist helped her develop a personalized exercise plan that gradually increased in intensity as she regained strength. The plan included a mix of aerobic exercises, strength training, and flexibility exercises.

Sarah discovered a passion for yoga, finding that it not only improved her physical flexibility but also provided mental and emotional benefits. Yoga became a daily practice, helping her manage stress and connect with her body in a mindful way.

In addition to yoga, Sarah enjoyed brisk walks in nature, swimming, and cycling. These activities allowed her to stay active while also spending time outdoors, which further boosted her mood and overall health.

One of the most significant changes Sarah made was prioritizing rest and recovery. She realized that her body needed time to heal and regenerate, and that meant getting enough sleep and allowing herself to rest when needed.

Sarah established a consistent sleep schedule, aiming for 7-8 hours of quality sleep each night. She created a relaxing bedtime routine that included reading, gentle stretching, and avoiding screens before bed. These changes improved her sleep quality, leaving her feeling more refreshed and energized each morning.

Managing Stress

Managing stress became a central focus in Sarah's new lifestyle. She understood that chronic stress could have detrimental effects on her health and recovery. Sarah explored various stress management techniques, including mindfulness meditation, deep breathing exercises, and journaling.

Mindfulness meditation helped Sarah stay present and reduce anxiety. She set aside time each day to practice meditation, finding that it calmed her mind and provided clarity. Journaling became a therapeutic outlet for her emotions, allowing her to process her experiences and express her thoughts.

Sarah's family played a crucial role in her adoption of a healthier lifestyle. James and the children joined her in making healthier choices, transforming their home environment into one that supported wellness. They started cooking meals together, engaging in physical activities as a family, and supporting each other's health goals.

The family also reduced their intake of processed foods and sugary snacks, opting for healthier alternatives. This collective effort created a supportive and encouraging atmosphere that made it easier for Sarah to stick to her new habits.

Regular Health Check-Ups

Sarah made it a priority to schedule regular health check-ups and follow-up appointments with her healthcare providers. These visits allowed her to monitor her progress, address any concerns, and make necessary adjustments to her lifestyle and treatment plan.

Her healthcare team, including her primary care physician, nutritionist, and physical therapist, provided valuable guidance and support. Regular check-ups ensured that Sarah stayed on track with her health goals and made informed decisions about her well-being.

Sarah recognized that her mental and emotional well-being was just as important as her physical health. She continued to attend counseling sessions, where she explored her thoughts and feelings in a safe and supportive environment. These sessions helped her build resilience and develop coping strategies for dealing with stress and anxiety.

In addition to professional support, Sarah leaned on her social network of friends and family. She made time for social activities that brought her joy and fulfillment, such as spending time with loved ones, participating in community events, and pursuing hobbies.

Mindfulness and gratitude became integral parts of Sarah's daily routine. She practiced mindfulness through meditation, yoga, and simply being present in the moment. This practice helped her stay grounded and focused on the positive aspects of her life.

Sarah also started a gratitude journal, where she recorded things she was thankful for each day. This practice shifted her perspective, allowing her to appreciate the small joys and victories in her recovery journey. It also helped her maintain a positive outlook and foster a sense of contentment.

Sarah's experience inspired her to become an advocate for health and wellness. She began sharing her story through local health awareness events, social media, and community talks. Sarah's goal was to raise awareness about septic shock, the importance of early detection, and the benefits of a healthy lifestyle.

Her advocacy efforts not only educated others but also provided her with a sense of purpose and fulfillment. Sarah found that helping others navigate their health challenges and inspiring them to make positive changes was incredibly rewarding.
Throughout her journey, Sarah learned the importance of setting realistic and achievable health goals. She celebrated small victories and acknowledged that progress might be slow but steady. This approach helped her stay motivated and

avoid feelings of frustration or discouragement.

Sarah set specific, measurable goals for her nutrition, exercise, and mental well-being. She tracked her progress and adjusted her goals as needed, allowing for flexibility and recognizing that setbacks were a natural part of the journey.

Sarah's commitment to a healthier lifestyle had a ripple effect on those around her. Her family, friends, and even colleagues were inspired by her transformation. Many of them began adopting healthier habits, creating a broader community of wellness.

Sarah's journey demonstrated the power of positive change and the impact one person's determination can have on others. Her story became a source of inspiration, motivating others to take charge of their health and make meaningful changes.

Chapter Six

Impact of her story on others and her role as an advocate

After surviving septic shock and embarking on a journey of recovery, Sarah felt a profound need to share her story. She believed that her experiences could offer hope, raise awareness, and potentially save lives. Sarah started by sharing her story with friends and family, but soon realized that her message could reach a broader audience.

The Power of Vulnerability

Sarah's willingness to be vulnerable and open about her struggles resonated deeply with others. She spoke candidly about the fear, pain, and uncertainty she faced during her illness and recovery. This honesty allowed people to connect with her on a personal level, understanding the profound impact septic shock had on her life.

Her story emphasized the importance of early detection and timely medical intervention. Sarah's narrative became a powerful tool in educating others about the signs and symptoms of sepsis, encouraging them to seek medical help without delay if they suspected an infection.

Sarah's advocacy began with local health awareness events. She volunteered to speak at community centers, schools, and hospitals, sharing her journey and highlighting the critical need for sepsis awareness. Her talks were well-received, and she quickly became a sought-after speaker for health-related events.

In her presentations, Sarah used her personal experiences to illustrate the broader message. She discussed the common signs of sepsis—such as high fever, rapid heart rate, confusion, and shortness of breath—and stressed the importance of recognizing these symptoms early. Her story served as a powerful reminder of the urgency required in treating sepsis.

Sarah also joined support groups for septic shock survivors, both online and offline. These groups provided a platform for her to connect with others who had similar experiences. She offered support, shared coping strategies, and listened to others' stories, creating a sense of community and mutual understanding.

Through these interactions, Sarah realized the importance of peer support in the recovery process. She became an active member of these groups, often leading discussions and organizing meet-ups. Her positive attitude and resilience inspired many, helping fellow survivors navigate their own recovery journeys.

Recognizing the power of social media, Sarah started a blog and social media accounts dedicated to raising awareness about sepsis and sharing health tips. Her posts included personal anecdotes, educational content, and resources for those affected by sepsis.

Sarah's online presence grew rapidly, attracting followers who were inspired by her story and motivated to learn more about sepsis. She collaborated with healthcare professionals to provide accurate information and partnered with organizations dedicated to sepsis awareness and prevention.

Sarah's efforts caught the attention of several healthcare organizations. She was invited to collaborate with these groups on awareness campaigns, educational programs, and advocacy initiatives. Sarah worked closely with sepsis foundations, hospitals, and public health agencies to spread her message.

One notable collaboration was with the Sepsis Alliance, a leading organization dedicated to raising sepsis awareness. Sarah participated in their campaigns, sharing her story through videos, articles, and public service announcements. Her involvement helped amplify the reach of these campaigns, educating thousands about sepsis prevention and early intervention.

Sarah also recognized the importance of educating healthcare providers about sepsis. She collaborated with medical professionals to develop training programs and workshops aimed at improving sepsis diagnosis and treatment. Sarah's firsthand experience provided valuable insights into the patient perspective, helping shape these educational initiatives.

She spoke at medical conferences, sharing her story with doctors, nurses, and medical students. Her presentations highlighted the importance of patient-centered care and the need for healthcare providers to listen to and trust their patients' concerns. Sarah's contributions helped bridge the gap between patients and healthcare professionals, fostering a more empathetic and responsive approach to sepsis care.

Sarah's advocacy extended to policy change as well. She joined forces with other advocates to lobby for improved sepsis protocols and funding for sepsis research. Sarah testified before legislative bodies, sharing her experience and emphasizing the need for greater awareness and resources to combat sepsis.

Her testimony was compelling, shedding light on the human impact of sepsis and the importance of early detection and treatment. Sarah's efforts contributed to increased funding for sepsis research and the development of national guidelines for sepsis management.
Sarah's story had a profound impact on individuals who heard or read about her experience. Many reached out to thank her for raising awareness and providing valuable information that had potentially saved lives. Sarah received messages from people who had recognized the symptoms of sepsis in themselves or their loved ones and sought medical help in time, thanks to her advocacy.

One particularly touching message came from a mother who had taken her child to the hospital after reading Sarah's story and recognizing the symptoms of sepsis. The child received timely treatment and made a full recovery. Stories like these reinforced Sarah's commitment to her advocacy work and highlighted the tangible impact of her efforts.

Sarah's advocacy created a lasting legacy of awareness, education, and support. Her journey from survivor to advocate inspired countless individuals to take charge of their health and stay informed about sepsis. Sarah's efforts contributed to a broader understanding of sepsis and improved outcomes for those affected by the condition.

As Sarah continued her advocacy, she remained dedicated to her mission of saving lives through education and awareness. Her story was a powerful reminder of the importance of resilience, community, and the impact one person can have on the lives of many.

Chapter Seven

Reflection on her Journey and the Lessons Learned

Sarah's journey from the brink of death to becoming a beacon of hope and advocate for sepsis awareness is a testament to the resilience of the human spirit. Reflecting on her journey, Sarah often marveled at how much her life had changed. What began as a terrifying ordeal transformed into an empowering mission that not only saved her life but also inspired and educated countless others.

The Power of Early Detection

One of the most profound lessons Sarah learned was the critical importance of early detection and treatment of sepsis. Her experience underscored the fact that timely medical intervention can mean the difference between life and death. This lesson became the cornerstone of her advocacy, driving her to educate others about the signs and symptoms of sepsis.

Resilience and Adaptability

Sarah's journey demonstrated the incredible resilience and adaptability of the human body and spirit. She endured immense physical and emotional challenges but continually found the strength to persevere.

Her recovery was not a straight path; it was filled with setbacks and difficulties. However, Sarah's ability to adapt to new circumstances, learn from her experiences, and maintain a positive outlook was crucial to her healing process.

The Importance of Support Systems

The support of Sarah's family, friends, and healthcare providers played an indispensable role in her recovery. Reflecting on her journey, Sarah realized how vital it was to have a strong support system. Their unwavering love, encouragement, and understanding helped her navigate the darkest moments and celebrate the milestones in her recovery.

Embracing Vulnerability

Sarah's willingness to share her story and be vulnerable was both challenging and transformative. She learned that opening up about her fears, struggles, and triumphs not only helped her heal but also created a deep connection with others. By embracing vulnerability, Sarah fostered empathy, understanding, and a sense of community among those who heard her story.

Finding Purpose in Adversity

The ordeal of septic shock gave Sarah a new sense of purpose. She realized that her experience could serve as a powerful tool for change. Instead of being defined by her illness, Sarah chose to use it as a platform to advocate for sepsis awareness and prevention. This newfound purpose gave her life deeper meaning and direction.

The Role of Self-Care

Sarah's journey highlighted the critical importance of self-care. Prior to her illness, she had often neglected her own needs in favor of her responsibilities and commitments. Her recovery taught her that taking care of herself—physically, mentally, and emotionally—was essential. Sarah learned to prioritize rest, nutrition, and mental well-being, understanding that self-care was not a luxury but a necessity.

Gratitude and Mindfulness

Throughout her recovery, Sarah cultivated a deep sense of gratitude and mindfulness. She learned to appreciate the small victories and the simple joys of life. Practicing mindfulness helped her stay present and focused on the positive aspects of her journey. Gratitude, in turn, provided her with a perspective that fostered resilience and contentment, even in the face of ongoing challenges.

The Impact of Advocacy

Sarah's advocacy efforts taught her about the profound impact one person can have. By sharing her story and educating others, she was able to raise awareness, influence healthcare practices, and potentially save lives. Sarah's journey demonstrated that even in the face of adversity, individuals have the power to effect meaningful change.

Strengthening Relationships

Sarah's experience brought her closer to her family and friends. The shared ordeal strengthened their bonds and deepened their understanding of one another. Sarah learned the importance of open communication, mutual support, and spending quality time with loved ones. These strengthened relationships became a source of joy and stability in her life.

Lifelong Learning

Sarah's journey was a continual process of learning and growth. She remained open to new information, willing to adapt her lifestyle, and eager to educate herself and others. This commitment to lifelong learning was essential in navigating her recovery and her role as an advocate. Sarah's experience underscored the value of staying informed and being proactive about health and wellness.

Empowerment Through Knowledge

Gaining knowledge about septic shock and the body's response to illness empowered Sarah. It enabled her to make informed decisions about her treatment and recovery. This empowerment extended to her advocacy work, where she aimed to provide others with the knowledge they needed to protect their health. Sarah's journey highlighted the transformative power of education and information.

Embracing Change

One of the most significant lessons Sarah learned was the importance of embracing change. Her life after septic shock was markedly different from before, but she chose to see these changes as opportunities for growth and improvement. Sarah adapted to her new reality with grace, finding new passions and purposes along the way.

The Value of Compassion

Sarah's experience deepened her compassion for others. She understood the pain and fear that come with serious illness and used this empathy to support and advocate for other patients. Sarah's journey taught her that compassion was not only a source of comfort for others but also a healing force for herself.

Looking Forward

Reflecting on her journey, Sarah felt a profound sense of accomplishment and hope. She had turned a life-threatening experience into a catalyst for positive change, not only for herself but for many others. Sarah looked forward to continuing her advocacy work, supporting septic shock survivors, and raising awareness about the importance of early detection and self-care.

About the Author

Hi, I am Dr. Jaylen Fleming. With over 10 years of clinical experience, I am a seasoned publisher dedicated to providing compassionate self-help resources on human health issues and diseases to patients and other health practitioners. Follow me for updates, and get my books to keep yourself enlightened and liberated.

Follow me on Amazon author central to get more of my books
https://www.amazon.com/author/drjaylen1

www.ingramcontent.com/pod-product-compliance
Lightning Source LLC
Chambersburg PA
CBHW071936210526
45479CB00002B/701